Pound droppers are winners

Recipes

*with max 10g fat
per meal*

Simone Margot

Pound droppers are winners

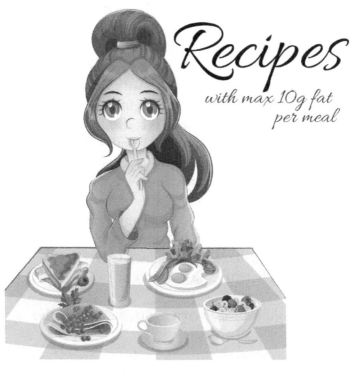

Recipes

*with max 10g fat
per meal*

Simone Margot

Copyright
Pound droppers are winners
Recipes
With max 10g fat per meal
Simone Margot
Cover Design: Arianny Garcia

ISBN: 9789083022987
NUR: 443
Printed by CreateSpace
Available on Kindle and other stores

Publisher:

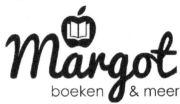

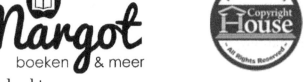

Zwijndrecht
The Netherlands

BREKFAST 13

LUNCH

BREAKFAST

APRICOT MUESLI

Serves: 1

Ingredients:
125g/4.4oz apricots
25g/1oz raspberries
40ml/1.5oz non-fat yoghurt
15g/1 tbsp oat flakes
15ml/1 tbsp lemon juice
22.5ml/1.5 tbsp liquid honey

Instructions:
1. Wash and slice the apricots and clean the raspberries.
2. Put this in a bowl and add half of the lemon juice and one tbsp of honey.
3. Let this rest for 5 minutes.
4. Mix the rest of the lemon juice and honey with the yoghurt.
5. Pour the yoghurt sauce over the fruit and sprinkle the oat flakes on top.

Nutritional info:
Calories: 190, Fat: 7g/1.4 tsp
Carbohydrates: 35g, Protein: 4g

BANANA MUESLI

Serves: 1

Ingredients:

50g/2oz raspberries
7.5g/0.5 tbsp hazelnuts
¼ papaya
1 banana

lemon juice
50g/3.5 tbsp yoghurt
5ml/1 tsp honey
15g/1 tbsp cornflakes

Instructions:
1. Put the hazelnuts in a pan to roast them; then chop them into little pieces.
2. Cut the papaya and the banana into little pieces. Add lemon juice on the papaya and banana.
3. Put the yoghurt in a bowl. Add the fruit, cornflakes and honey.
4. Top the dish with the roasted nuts.

Nutritional info:
Calories: 280, Fat: 6g/1.2 tsp
Carbohydrates:: 48g, Protein: 6g

BELL PEPPER CRISPBREAD

Serves: 1

Ingredients:
1 bell pepper
3 slices whole wheat crispbread
50g/3 tbsp cream cheese
salt
pepper
2 stems chive

Instructions:
1. Cut the bell pepper into little cubes.
2. Smear the crispbread with the cream cheese.
3. Sprinkle the bell pepper cubes on top.
4. Season with salt and pepper.
5. Roll up the chives and finely chop the roll.
6. Sprinkle these rolls on top of the crispbread.

Nutritional info:
Calories: 250, Fat: 9g/1.8 tsp
Carbohydrates: 22g, Protein: 9g

BLUEBERRY MIX

Serves: 1

Ingredients:
100g/3.5oz blueberries
200g/7oz cottage cheese
30g/2 tbsp quinoa

Instructions:
1. Stir the blueberries in the cottage cheese.
2. Pop the quinoa in a pan.
3. Add the popped quinoa on top.

Nutritional info:
Calories: 205, Fat: 3g/0.6 tsp
Carbohydrates: 16g, Protein: 28g

BREAKFAST ROLLS

Serves: 1

Ingredients:
2 spring onions
100g/3.5oz low-fat cottage cheese
4 slices boiled ham
4 leaves chicory

Instructions:
1. Cut the spring onion into little pieces.
2. Wash the chicory leaves and dry.
3. Mix the spring onion with the cottage cheese.
4. Take a slice of ham and put a chicory leaf on it.
5. Add one quarter the onion-cheese mixture and roll up the ham.

Nutritional info:
Calories: 250, Fat: 4g/0.8 tsp
Carbohydrates: 10g, Protein: 37g

CAMEMBERT TOAST

Serves: 1

Ingredients:
1 slice whole-wheat bread
30g/2 tbsp low-fat cream cheese
2.5g/0.5 tsp tomato puree
100g/7 tbsp cucumber
60g/4 tbsp camembert/maximum of 13g fat

Instructions:
1. Roast the bread.
2. Mix the cream cheese with the tomato puree and smear on the bread.
3. Slice the cucumber.
4. Cut the camembert into cubes.
5. Add the camembert and cucumber slices on top.

Nutritional info:
Calories: 230, Fat: 6g/1.2 tsp
Carbohydrates: 6g, Protein: 21g

CHICKEN BREAST SANDWICHES

Serves: 1

Ingredients:
2 whole-wheat slices of bread
30g/2 tbsp low-fat cottage cheese
0.5 apricot
3 slices of chicken breast

Instructions:
1. Smear both bread slices with the cottage cheese.
2. Slice the apricot.
3. Add the chicken breast and apricot on top.

Nutritional info:
Calories: 200, Fat: 1g/0.2 tsp
Carbohydrates: 29g, Protein: 16g

CHOCOLATE COTTAGE CHEESE

Serves: 1

Ingredients:
250g/9oz cottage cheese
15g/1 tbsp chocolate powder
5ml/1 tsp honey
the marrow of a half vanilla stem
1 banana

Instructions:
1. Put the cottage cheese in a bowl.
2. Add the chocolate powder, the honey and the marrow.
3. Slice the banana and garnish the cottage cheese mixture.

Nutritional info:
Calories: 340, Fat: 3g/0.6 tsp
Carbohydrates: 40g, Protein: 37g

CHEESE RAISIN SANDWICH

Serves: 1

Ingredients:
45g/3 tbsp rosehip sauce
the marrow of a quarter vanilla stem
3 slices raisin bread
80g/3oz cream cheese

Instructions:
1. Mix the rosehip sauce with the marrow.
2. Smear the raisin bread with the cream cheese.
3. Add the rosehip sauce on top.

Nutritional info:
Calories: 410, Fat: 9g/1.8 tsp
Carbohydrates: 60g, Protein: 15g

CHICKEN TOAST

Serves: 1

Ingredients:
Chicken toast
2 slices whole-grain toast bread
2 slices chicken breast filet
20g/4 tsp low-fat cream cheese
15g/1 tbsp chives

Smoothie
75g/3oz sugar melon
75g/3oz non-fat yoghurt
fresh peppermint by choice

Instructions:
Chicken toast
1. Toast the bread until golden brown and let them cool off.
2. Put on one slice the chicken breast filet.
3. Cut the chives.
4. Put on the other bread, slice the cream cheese and sprinkle the cut chives on top.

Smoothie
1. Puree the flesh of the melon with the yoghurt.
2. Decorate with fresh peppermint.

Nutritional info:
Calories: 200, Fat: 3g/0.6 tsp
Carbohydrates: 30g, Protein: 12g

EGG SANDWICH

Serves: 1

Ingredients:

1 egg
30ml/2 tbsp low-fat yoghurt
mustard
salt
pepper

0.5 bunch of chives
5g/1 tsp cashews
1 slice whole-grain bread
1 tomato

Instructions:

1. Boil the egg until hard, cool off and peel.
2. Chop the peeled egg and put in a bowl.
3. Add the yoghurt, mustard, salt and pepper with the egg.
4. Chop the bunch of chives and the cashews.
5. Add to the egg salad.
6. Put the salad on a slice of bread.
7. Slice the tomato and garnish the slice of bread.

Nutritional info:

Calories: 200, Fat: 9g/1.8 tsp
Carbohydrates: 18g, Protein: 12g

FILLED GRAPEFRUIT

Serves: 1

Ingredients:
0.5 pink grapefruit
1 stem mint
150g/5oz low-fat cream cheese
2.5ml/0.5 tsp honey

Instructions:
1. Remove the wedges from the grapefruit.
2. Cut the mint in stripes.
3. Mix the cream cheese with the honey.
4. Add the grapefruit wedges and mix.
5. Fill the zest from the grapefruit with the cheese mixture.

Nutritional info:
Calories: 150, Fat: 2g/0.4 tsp
Carbohydrates: 15g, Protein: 21g

FRUIT COTTAGE CHEESE BOWL

Serves: 1

Ingredients:
6 apricot halves
50g/3.5 tbsp grapes
200g/7oz non-fat cottage cheese
30ml/2 tbsp non-fat milk
5ml/1 tsp lemon juice

Instructions:
1. Slice the apricot halves.
2. Rinse the grapes and slice them in halves.
3. Put the cottage cheese in a bowl.
4. Add the milk and the lemon juice and stir until the mixture is smooth.
5. Stir in almost all the fruit.
6. Decorate the bowl with the small rest of the fruit.

Nutritional info:
Calories: 179, Fat: 1g/0.2 tsp
Carbohydrates: 12g, Protein: 28g

FRUIT RICE

Serves: 1

Ingredients:
50g/2oz Basmati rice
50 ml/2oz apple juice
5ml/1 tsp liquid honey
150g/ 5oz non-fat yoghurt
1 kiwi
150g/5oz strawberries

Instructions:
1. Cook the rice according to the description on the package and let the rice cool off.
2. Add the apple juice and the honey to the yoghurt and stir until you have a creamy mass.
3. Cut the kiwi and the strawberries into bite-sized chunks.
4. Stir the yoghurt creme through the cold rice. Put this on a plate and put the fruit on top.

Nutritional info:
Calories: 380, Fat: 5g/1 tsp
Carbohydrates: 70g, Protein: 15g

HAM CARPACCIO

Serves: 1

Ingredients:

150g/5oz blue grapes
1 small apple
75g/3oz low-fat yoghurt
20g/4 tsp low-fat cream cheese

5g/1 tsp mustard
salt
pepper
100g/3.5oz boiled ham

Instructions:

1. Cut the grapes into halves and slice the apple.
2. Put the yoghurt in a bowl.
3. Add the cream cheese and mustard and stir.
4. Season with salt and pepper.
5. Spread the ham slices on a plate.
6. Garnish with the apple slices and grape halves.
7. Pour the sauce on top.

Nutritional info:
Calories: 315, Fat: 3g/0.6 tsp
Carbohydrates: 43g, Protein: 29g

HAM MELON ROLL

Serves: 1

Ingredients:
1 whole-wheat roll
10g/2 tsp half-fat butter
15g/1 tbsp low-fat ham/max 3%
150g/5oz sugar melon flesh

Instructions:
1. Cut the roll into halves.
2. Smear the butter onto the halves.
3. Add the ham.
4. Slice the melon flesh.
5. Garnish the melon slices on top of the ham.

Nutritional info:
Calories: 215, Fat: 5g/1 tsp
Carbohydrates: 34g, Protein: 8g

HERBAL SCRAMBLED EGGS

Serves: 1

Ingredients:

1 tomato   1 egg
1 spring onion   salt
15ml/1 tbsp oil   pepper
2 stems parsley   1 slice white bread
2 stems dill

Instructions:
1. Cut the tomato and spring onion into little pieces.
2. Take a pan to heat the oil and add the tomato and onion and roast both.
3. Finely chop the parsley and dill. Beat the egg also, mix in the herbs.
4. Put the egg in the pan with the tomato and onion.
5. Season with salt and pepper.
6. Bake everything until well done and put it on the bread slice.

Nutritional info:
Calories: 120, Fat: 6g/1.2 tsp
Carbohydrates: 20g, Protein: 12g

MELON FLAKES

Serves: 1

Ingredients:
200g/7oz watermelon/without peel and kernels
200 ml/7oz non-fat yoghurt
15ml/1 tbsp lemon juice
5ml/1 tsp liquid honey
20g/4 tsp sugar-free cornflakes

Instructions:
1. Cut the watermelon into cubes.
2. Put the yoghurt in a bowl. Stir in the lemon juice and honey.
3. Add the melon and cornflakes in the bowl and mix.

Nutritional info:
Calories: 290, Fat: 7g/1.4 tsp
Carbohydrates: 46g, Protein: 10g

MELON MUESLI

Serves: 1

Ingredients:
3 tbsp oat flakes
5 tbsp milk
200g/7oz watermelon without peel and kernels
100 ml/3.5oz yoghurt
lemon juice
vanilla powder

Instructions:
1. Put the oat flakes in a bowl and pour the milk on top.
2. Let this soak briefly.
3. Cut the watermelon into bite-sized pieces and mix this with the oat flakes.
4. Mix the yoghurt with a little lemon juice and vanilla powder.
5. Put this on top of the oatmeal mixture.

Nutritional info:
Calories: 280, Fat: 4g/0.8 tsp
Carbohydrates: 49g, Protein: 13g

OAT MUESLI

Serves: 1

Ingredients:
30g/2 tbsp oat flakes
1 orange
150 ml/5oz non-fat yoghurt
cinnamon

Instructions:
1. Roast the oat flakes in a non-stick pan without fat.
2. Cut the flesh of the orange in little cubes.
3. Mix these cubes with the yoghurt.
4. Sprinkle the oat flakes and some cinnamon on top.

Nutritional info:
Calories: 220, Fat: 4g/0.8 tsp,
Carbohydrates: 34g, Protein: 12g

OATMEAL WITH FRUIT

Serves: 1

Ingredients:
250 ml/9oz milk
50g/3.5 tbsp oats
5ml/1 tsp lemon juice
1 peach
50g/3.5 tbsp strawberries

Instructions:
1. Boil the milk and gradually add the oats. Stir in the lemon juice.
2. Cook the oats until they are thick enough.
3. Cut the peach and strawberries into cubes.
4. Put the fruit cubes on top.

Nutritional info:
Calories: 390, Fat: 8g/1.6 tsp
Carbohydrates: 54g, Protein: 16g

ORANGE COTTAGE CHEESE

Serves: 1

Ingredients:
100g/3.5oz raspberries
1 orange
150g/5oz cottage cheese

Instructions:
1. Wash the raspberries.
2. Divide the orange into loose parts and save the orange juice.
3. Mix the orange juice with the cottage cheese.
4. Put the orange parts and raspberries in a bowl.
5. Add the cottage cheese on top.

Nutritional info:
Calories: 220, Fat: 2g/0.4 tsp
Carbohydrates: 16g, Protein: 24g,

PAPAYA PUMPERNICKEL BREAD

Serves: 1

Ingredients:
0.5 medium-size papaya
60ml/4 tbsp non-fat yoghurt
1 slice of pumpernickel bread

Instructions:
1. Slice the flesh of the papaya and arrange them in a soup plate.
2. Pour the yoghurt on the papaya and crumble the pumpernickel bread on top.

Nutritional info:
Calories: 180, Fat: 2g/0.4 tsp
Carbohydrates: 34g, Protein: 7g

PEAR TOAST

Serves: 1

Ingredients:
2 slices of brown bread
60g/4 tbsp cottage cheese
1 pear
10g/2 tsp cranberries/jar

Instructions:
1. Toast the bread.
2. Smear the cottage cheese on the toast.
3. Peel the pear and slice the pear.
4. Divide the slices onto the toast.
5. Garnish with the cranberries.

Nutritional info:
Calories: 330, Fat: 4g/0.8 tsp
Carbohydrates: 52gProtein: 18g

PORRIDGE

Serves:1

Ingredients:
60g/4 tbsp oat flakes
150 ml/5oz non-fat milk
45g/3 tbsp cranberries
5 ml/1 tsp honey
50g/3.5 tbsp frozen blueberries

Instructions:
1. Roast the oat flakes in a non-stick pan.
2. Add the milk and cranberries in the pan.
3. Let this simmer until thoroughly warm.
4. Season with the honey.
5. Add the blueberries.

Nutritional info:
Calories: 290, Fat: 5g/1 tsp
Carbohydrates: 40g, Protein: 9g,

RASPBERRY SHAKE

Serves: 1

Ingredients:
150g/5oz raspberries
300 ml/10oz kefir or yoghurt
15g/1 tbsp of oat flakes

Instructions:
1. Mix the raspberries with the kefir and puree.
2. Put this mixture in a bowl.
3. Add the oat flakes on top.

Nutritional info:
Calories: 220, Fat: 6g/1.2 tsp
Carbohydrates: 27g, Protein: 14g,

ROASTED BUN WITH PEACHES

Serves: 1

Ingredients:

1 peach or two apricots
5ml/1 tsp honey
lime juice

1 white roll
30g/2 tbsp ricotta

Instructions:

1. Immerse the peach or the apricots in boiling water, scare with cold water and peel. Cut the fruit into wedges.
2. Put the slices in a pan together with the honey and a little lime juice.
3. Heat the pan and heat the slices until they are warm. Then take the pan off the fire.
4. Cut the roll in half and grill the halves until they are brittle.
5. Spread each half with one tbsp ricotta and put half of the peach or apricot slices on top.

Nutritional info:

Calories: 220, Fat: 1g/0.2 tsp
Carbohydrates: 50g, Protein: 6g,

SALMON ROLL

Serves: 1

Ingredients:
5g/1 tsp horseradish
50g/2oz non-fat cottage cheese
1 whole-wheat roll
60g/2.5oz salmon
300g/10oz watermelon /no peel and seeds

Instructions:
1. Add the horseradish to the cottage cheese and stir until creamy.
2. Cut the roll into halves and smear both halves with the cream.
3. Divide the salmon on top of the creamy halves.
4. Gently roll-up.
5. Cut the watermelon into bite-sized chunks.
6. Take a big plate and garnish it all.

Nutritional info:
Calories: 380, Fat: 5g/1 tsp
Carbohydrates: 58g, Protein: 26g,

SANDWICH CHEESE KIWI

Serves: 1

Ingredients:
1 kiwi
100g/3.5oz strawberries
2 slices of whole wheat bread
60g/4 tbsp of cottage cheese
10g/2 tsp of honey

Instructions:
1. Slice the kiwi and the strawberries.
2. Smear each slice of bread with two tbsp of cottage cheese and one tsp of honey.
3. Divide the kiwi and strawberries on top.

Nutritional info:
Calories: 390, Fat: 7g/1.4 tsp
Carbohydrates: 56g, Protein: 22g,

PINEAPPLE SMOOTHIE

Serves: 1

Ingredients:
1 peach
150g/5oz pineapple chunks
20g/2 tbsp baby spinach
5g/1 tsp grated ginger
60ml/4 tbsp water
10g/2 tsp coconut grate

Instructions:
1. Submerge the peach in hot water to remove the skin.
2. Cut the fruit flesh into cubes.
3. Put the pineapple chunks, spinach, peach, ginger, water and coconut grate in a blender and mix.

Nutritional info:
Calories: 140, Fat: 8g/1.6 tsp
Carbohydrates: 14g, Protein: 2g

STRAWBERRY BREAKFAST

Serves: 1

Ingredients:
250g/9oz strawberries
250 ml/9oz non-fat yoghurt
200 ml/7oz non-fat milk
10g/2 tsp sugar
1 package vanilla sugar

Instructions:
1. Cut half of the strawberries into halves and sprinkle the sugar on top.
2. Puree the rest of the strawberries with the vanilla sugar.
3. Mix the puree with the yoghurt and milk.
4. Put this mixture in a bowl and decorate with the sugared strawberries.

Nutritional info:
Calories: 340, Fat: 4g/0.8 tsp
Carbohydrates: 50g, Protein: 20g

STRAWBERRY FLAKE

Serves: 1

Ingredients:
100g/3.5oz strawberries
15g/1 tbsp grated almonds
30g/2 tbsp cornflakes
100 ml/3.5oz milk

Instructions:
1. Cut the strawberries into quarters.
2. Put the almonds in a pan without fat to roast.
3. Put the cornflakes in a dish and add the milk.
4. Add the strawberries and almonds on top.

Nutritional info:
Calories: 220, Fat: 5g/1 tsp
Carbohydrates: 36g, Protein: 8g

STRAWBERRY MUESLI DRINK

Serves: 1

Ingredients:
150g/5oz defrosted strawberries
30g/2 tbsp non-fat yoghurt
150 ml/5oz non-fat milk
1.2g/0.25 tsp vanilla sugar
30g/2 tbsp soft oat flakes

Instructions:
1. Put the strawberries in a blender, or a large bowl for the mixer.
2. Add the yoghurt, milk, vanilla sugar and oat flakes.
3. Blend everything or use the mixer with the purer bar.
4. Pour in a glass.

Nutritional info:
Calories: 240, Fat: 5g/1 tsp
Carbohydrates: 32g, Protein: 12g

TOAST WITH ROAST BEEF

Serves: 1

Ingredients:
4 radishes
4 slices roast beef
1 slice whole-wheat bread
10g/2 tsp horseradish
10g/2 tsp non-fat cottage cheese

Instructions:
1. Cut the radishes into small cubes.
2. Put the roast beef slices on a tray and sprinkle the radish cubes on top.
3. Roll up the roast beef slices.
4. Toast the bread until golden brown.
5. Blend the horseradish with the cottage cheese and smear on the bread.
6. Garnish with the roast beef rolls.

Nutritional info:
Calories: 250, Fat: 8g/1.6 tsp
Carbohydrates: 17g, Protein: 28g

TOMATO SANDWICH

Serves: 1

Ingredients:
2 slices whole-wheat bread
30g/2 tbsp ricotta
6 tomato slices
various herbs

Instructions:
1. Smear the ricotta on the bread.
2. Divide the tomato slices on top.
3. Add herbs for flavour.

Nutritional info:
Calories: 310, Fat: 8g.1.6 tsp
Carbohydrates: 41g, Protein: 18g

SALMON CRISPBREAD

Serves: 1

Ingredients:
2 crispbread
150g/5oz cottage cheese
8 pickles
6 salmon slices

Instructions:
1. Smear each crispbread with the cottage cheese.
2. Put on each crispbread three salmon slices
3. Dice the pickles and sprinkle on top

Nutritional info:
Calories: 230, Fat: 2g/0.4 tsp
Carbohydrates: 16g, Protein: 37g

VEGETABLE GRATE

Serves: 1

Ingredients:
1 small cucumber
1 small carrot
30g/2 tbsp mineral water
50g/2oz soft curd cheese
salt
pepper
2 slices whole wheat crispbread

Instructions:
1. Peel the cucumber and cut the cucumber in half lengthwise.
2. Cut out the core and grate the rest.
3. Peel the carrot and grate it.
4. Mix the mineral water with the curd cheese.
5. Stir in the grated cucumber and carrot also, season with salt and pepper.
6. Divide the mixture over the crispbread.

Nutritional info:
Calories: 140, Fat: 1g/0.2 tsp
Carbohydrates: 22g, Protein: 11g

BANANA SANDWICH

Serves: 1

Ingredients:
30g/2 tbsp cream cheese
1 slice whole-wheat bread
15g/1 tbsp plum sauce
80g/3oz banana

Instructions:
1. Smear the cream cheese onto the bread.
2. Put the plum sauce on top.
3. Slice the banana and add on top of the plum sauce.

Nutritional info:
Calories: 235, Fat: 1g/0.2 tsp
Carbohydrates: 43g, Protein: 9g

CAMEMBERT AND RASPBERRIES

Serves: 1

Ingredients:
1 small piece camembert/13-g fat
2 slices whole-wheat bread
10 raspberries

Instructions:
1. Slice the camembert piece.
2. Put the slices on the bread.
3. Mash the raspberries with a fork and put them on top of the camembert bread.

Nutritional info:
Calories: 225, Fat: 8g/1.6 tsp
Carbohydrates: 20g, Protein: 18g

YOGHURT DUTCH RUSK DREAM

Serves: 1

Ingredients:
15g/1 tbsp sesame seed
25g/2 tbsp walnuts
2 Dutch rusk biscuits
200g/7oz Greek yoghurt
5g/1 tsp liquid honey

Instructions:
1. Roast the sesame seed in a non-stick frying pan.
2. Chop the walnuts and crumble the Dutch rusk biscuits in big pieces.
3. Take a bowl and fill it with the yoghurt.
4. Sprinkle the sesame seed, walnuts and the biscuits on top.
5. Drizzle the honey over the mixture.

Nutritional info:
Calories: 310, Fat: 10g/2 tsp
Carbohydrates: 30g, Protein: 24

LUNCH

SPICY BEANS WITH BEEF

Serves: 1

Ingredients:
1 onion
5ml/1 tsp oil
100g/3.5oz low-fat beef
150g/5oz tomato chunks
salt
cayenne pepper
50 ml/5 tbsp instant vegetable broth
5g/1 tsp tomato paste
100g/3.5oz big white beans/canned
2 stems parsley chopped

Instructions:
1. Dice the onion and heat the oil in a non-stick pan.
2. Add the onion and beef and bake the beef crumble.
3. Add the tomato chunks. Season with salt and cayenne pepper and add the vegetable broth. Recook everything. Add the tomato paste.
4. Rinse the beans and put them in the pan.
5. Recook until everything is well done.
6. Finely chop the parsley.
7. Put on a plate and sprinkle parsley on top.

Nutritional info:
Calories: 290, Fat: 10g /2 tsp
Carbohydrate 30g, Protein: 30g

MUSHROOM PASTA WITH HAM

Serves: 1

Ingredients:
50g/2oz whole wheat pasta
2 spring onions
100g/3.5oz mushrooms
20g/1oz low-fat ham
50ml/3 tbsp instant vegetable broth
15ml/1 tbsp cooking cream

Instructions:

1. Cook the pasta as mentioned on the package.
2. Cut the spring onion into rings and slice the mushrooms.
3. Cut the ham into cubes.
4. Take a non-stick frying pan and add the oil. Fry the ham cubes, mushrooms and spring onions until they are brown.
5. Add the broth and cooking cream and recook for a few seconds.
6. Rinse the pasta and add to the pan—season with salt and pepper. Sprinkle chopped parsley on top.

Nutritional info:

Calories: 300, Fat: 9g/1.8 tsp
Carbohydrate: 40g, Protein: 14g

BELL PEPPER RICE

Serves: 1

Ingredients
30g/2 tbsp whole wheat rice
100g/3.5oz chicken fillet
5ml/1 tsp oil
1 red bell pepper
100ml/3.5oz water
salt
chilli powder
parsley

Instructions

1. Cook the rice as described on the package.
2. Cut the chicken fillet into strips.
3. Heat the oil in a non-stick pan and bake the meat.
4. Cut the bell pepper into little cubes and add to the meat.
5. Bake the cubes for a short time with the meat and add the water to cool off the pan and let everything simmer till done.
6. Season the mix with salt and chilli powder.
7. Add the rice, mix everything and serve with chopped parsley.

Nutritional info:
Calories: 340, Fat: 8g/1.6 tsp
Carbohydrate: 39g, Protein: 30g

CHICKEN BOWL

Serves: 1

Ingredients
60g/2oz whole-grain rice
0.25 medium-sized eggplant
1 clove garlic
150g/5oz chicken fillet
2 spring onions
1 stem thyme
5ml/1 tsp oil
2.5g/0.5 tsp curry
1 knife tip coriander powder
5g/1 tsp mustard seed
1 chilli
125ml/4.5oz chicken broth
salt
pepper
150g/5oz frozen pumpkin cubes

Instructions

1. Cook the rice as described on the package.
2. Cut the eggplant, garlic, chicken fillet and spring onion into cubes.
3. Roughly chop the thyme.
4. Take a pan and heat the oil. Add the chicken fillet and bake until the meat is medium brown.
5. Add the vegetables, garlic, herbs and chilli and cook everything well done. Add the broth and season.
6. Let this simmer until everything is well cooked.
7. Add the frozen pumpkin cubes and recook— season with salt and pepper.

Nutritional info:
Calories: 490, Fat: 7g/1.4 tsp
Carbohydrate:67g, Protein: 42g

EGG AND CORN SALAD

Serves: 1

Ingredients:
1 egg
1 apple
lemon juice
2 pickles
2 spring onions
1 small red bell pepper
70g/2.5oz little can corn
100ml/3.5oz low-fat yoghurt
paprika
salt
pepper
parsley

Instructions:
1. Boil the egg until hard.
2. Cut the apple into small chunks and drizzle a little bit of lemon juice on top.
3. Slice the pickles and cut the spring onions in rings.
4. Cut the bell pepper in cubes.
5. Drain the corn.
6. Mix everything in a bowl.
7. Take another bowl for the yoghurt. Mix the yoghurt with lemon juice, paprika, salt and pepper.
8. Pour this sauce over the vegetables.
9. Slice the egg in four pieces and put on top of the salad.
10. Sprinkle parsley on top.

Nutritional info:
Calories: 300, Fat: 9g/1.8 tsp
Carbohydrate: 38g, Protein: 16g

APPLE WITH KOHLRABI AND HAM

Serves: 1

Ingredients:
1 small kohlrabi
0.5 yellow bell pepper
1 apple
I pickle
3 stems dill
100g/3.5oz low-fat yoghurt
5ml/1 tsp lemon juice
5ml/1 tsp oil
1 romaine lettuce
50g/2oz boiled ham

Instructions:
1. Cut the kohlrabi, bell pepper, apple and pickle into same-sized cubes and put them in a bowl.
2. Finely cut the dill.
3. Put the yoghurt in a dish. Add the lemon juice, oil and dill and stir into a creamy sauce.
4. Pour the sauce over the cubes and mix everything. Let this soak for about 20 minutes.
5. Remove the leaves from the lettuce, wash and dry them.
6. Cut the ham into strips.
7. Add the mixed vegetable salad and sprinkle the ham stripes on top.

Nutritional info:
Calories: 290, Fat: 9g/1.8 tsp
Carbohydrate: 32g, Protein: 20g

POTATO CABBAGE SALAD

Serves: 1

Ingredients:
150g/5.5oz potatoes
125g/4.5oz savoy
50 ml/2oz vegetable broth
15ml/1 tbsp vinegar
5g/1 tsp mustard
60g/4 tbsp mushrooms
5ml/1 tsp oil
5 radishes
2 stems parsley
salt
pepper

Instructions:

1. Cook the potatoes well done for about 20 minutes. Peel and slice them and put them in a bowl.
2. Boil some water in a second pan and add a little bit of salt.
3. Cut the cabbage in stripes and parboil them for 3-4 minutes in the saltwater.
4. Let the stripes dry up in a colander.
5. Cook the vegetable broth in a saucepan and take the saucepan off the fire.
6. Add vinegar and mustard and pour this mixture over the potato slices.
7. Let this mixture cool off and come to taste for about 20 minutes
8. Cut the mushrooms in halves. Heat the oil in a pan and bake the mushrooms.
9. Slice the radishes and finely cut the parsley.
10. Mix the cabbage, mushrooms, radishes and parsley with the potato slices.
11. Season, if necessary, with salt and pepper.

Nutritional info:
Calories: 150, Fat: 4g/0.8 tsp
Carbohydrate: 20g, Protein: 8g

PINEAPPLE SALAD

Serves 1

Ingredients:
100g/3.5oz pineapple chunks
0.25 pomegranate
lime juice
25g/2 tbsp full-fat yoghurt
1.2g/0.25 tbsp honey
salt

Instructions:
1. Remove the seeds from the pomegranate by hitting the skin.
2. Put the pineapple chunks in a dish. Sprinkle the seeds on top.
3. Add a little lime juice to the yoghurt, honey and a pinch of salt.
4. Pour the sauce on top of the fruit in the dish.

Nutritional info:
Calories: 130, Fat: 4g/0.8 tsp
Carbohydrate: 19g, Protein: 3g

BAGUETTE WITH SALMON

Serves 1

Ingredients:
1 small cucumber
lemon juice
40g/2.5 tbsp low-fat cream cheese
1 shallot
1 whole-wheat baguette roll
40g/2.5 tbsp smoked salmon

Instructions:
1. Grate the cucumber. Mix this with the cream cheese and add some lemon juice.
2. Finely dice the shallot.
3. Cut the baguette in half and besmear each of the halve with the cream cheese mixture.
4. Sprinkle the chopped onion on top.
5. Add the salmon on top. Put the other half of the baguette roll on top.

Nutritional info:
Calories: 365, Fat: 4g/0.8 tsp
Carbohydrate: 60g, Protein: 21g

BULGUR SALAD WITH TOMATOES

Serves: 1

Ingredients:
40g/2.5 tbsp bulgur
10g/1 tbsp pine nuts
50g/2oz cherry tomatoes
0.5 cucumber
1 stem mint
1 stem coriander
1 stem parsley
10 raisins
0.25 lemon
5ml/1 tsp olive oil
salt
pepper

Instructions:

1. Cook the bulgur as mentioned on the package.
2. Roast the pine nuts and put them in a bowl to cool off.
3. Cut the tomatoes in four pieces. Cut the cucumber into little cubes.
4. Chop the mint, coriander and parsley.
5. Put the bulgur in a bowl and add the pine pits
6. Add the tomatoes, cucumber, raisins and chopped herbs.
7. Squeeze the lemon and add the juice to the olive oil.
8. Season with salt and pepper to taste.
9. Stir everything in the bulgur and, if necessary, season with salt and pepper.

Nutritional info:

Calories: 160, Fat: 6g/1.2 tsp
Carbohydrate: 20g, Protein: 5g

WATERMELON BULGUR SALAD

Serves 1

Ingredients:
40g/2.5 tbsp bulgur
1 small cucumber
100ml/3.5oz Greek yoghurt
1 garlic clove
salt
pepper
300g/10.5oz watermelon/no peel and kernels
3 stems parsley
30ml/2 tbsp lemon juice
5ml/1 tsp oil

Instructions:
1. Cook the bulgur as described on the package and loosen with a fork.
2. Peel the cucumber, remove the core and grate with a grate.
3. Mix this with the yoghurt. Press the garlic clove and stir into the yoghurt.
4. Season with salt and pepper.
5. Cut the watermelon into little cubes. Finely chop the parsley.
6. Mix the melon with the parsley, lemon juice and oil through the bulgur.
7. Leave to soak for about 15 minutes.
8. Put this on a plate and add the yoghurt dip on top.

Nutritional info:
Calories: 365, Fat: 7g/1.4 tsp
Carbohydrate: 56g, Protein: 18g

COLD MELON GINGER SOUP

Serves: 1

Ingredients:
0.5 melon
1 small piece of ginger
200 ml/7oz non-fat yoghurt
5ml/1 tsp lemon juice
salt
pepper

Instructions:
1. Remove most of the fruit flesh from the melon with a spoon. Leave a rim of fruit flesh.
2. Peel the ginger and slice the ginger in tiny cubes.
3. Mix the fruit flesh, ginger, yoghurt and lime juice and puree.
4. Season with salt and pepper.
5. Pour the mixture in the melon and store it in the fridge for about one hour.

Nutritional info:
Calories: 210, Fat: 8g/1.6 tsp
Carbohydrate: 25g, Protein: 8g

CURRY RICE SALAD WITH MELON

Serves 1

Ingredients:

40g/1.50z brown rice
100ml/3.50z non-fat
yoghurt
salt
pepper
mild curry powder
0.5 garlic clove

150g/5.50z cherry
tomatoes
50g/3 tbsp pees
1 small pear
150g/5.50z watermelon
fruit flesh

Instructions:

1. Cook the rice as described on the package and let it cool off quickly.
2. Put the yoghurt in a bowl and mix with the salt, pepper and curry powder.
3. Chop the garlic and cut the cherry tomatoes in halves. Blanch the peas and cut the pear into little chunks. Mix the garlic, tomatoes, peas and pear chunks and leave to infuse.
4. Take the cold rice and add the infused mix.
5. Cut the melon flesh into little cubes, and serve.

Nutritional info:

Calories: 300, Fat: 2g/0.4 tsp
Carbohydrate: 59g, Protein: 12g

CURRY RICE SALAD

Serves 1

Ingredients:
50g/3 tbsp rice
1 small red bell pepper
1 carrot
1 apple
150ml/5oz yoghurt
lemon juice
2.5g/0.5 tsp curry powder
pepper
salt

Instructions:

1. Cook the rice as mentioned on the package, pour the rice and allow to cool quickly.
2. Cut the bell pepper into little cubes. Slice the carrot and apple.
3. Add a little lemon juice on the apple slices. Mix this into the rice.
4. Stir the curry powder, pepper and salt through the yoghurt.
5. Put the rice on a plate and garnish with the yoghurt.

Nutritional info:
Calories: 370, Fat: 4g/0.8 tsp
Carbohydrate: 69g, Protein: 15g

FRUIT SALAD WITH YOGHURT DIP

Serves 1

Ingredients:
50g/2oz blueberries
50g/2oz raspberries
0.5 apple
1 peach
0.5 banana
0.13 pineapple
0.13 pomegranate

Dip
40ml/3 tbsp full-fat yoghurt
Some maple syrup
Some orange juice

Instructions:
1. Wash the blueberries and the raspberries.
2. Remove the core from the apple and the peach and slice both in
3. Slice the banana and drizzle the slices with some lemon juice.
4. Cut the pineapple into bite-sized chunks
5. Hit the pomegranate to loosen the kernels.
6. Put all the fruit in a bowl and pour the dip on top.

Dip
1. Put the yoghurt in a small bowl.
2. Stir in maple syrup and orange juice to taste.

Nutritional info:
Calories: 220, Fat: 2g /0.4 tsp
Carbohydrate: 43g, Protein: 3g

SHRIMPS ON A CARROT SALAD

Serves: 1

Ingredients:
150g/5.3oz carrots
15ml/1 tsp olive oil
some vanilla marrow
5ml/1 tsp lemon juice
2.5ml/0.5 tsp olive oil
salt
pepper
60g/4 tbsp frozen shrimps
1 beetroot

Instructions:

1. Heat one teaspoon of olive oil in a saucepan and add a little vanilla marrow.
2. When thoroughly mixed, let it simmer.
3. Grate the carrots and the beetroot. When finished, take the vanilla oil off the heat source and let it cool off.
4. Mix one tsp of lemon juice with the halve tsp of olive oil—season with salt and pepper.
5. Defrost the shrimps and peel on to the tale, remove the colon with a knife.
6. Heat a tsp of olive oil in a saucepan and bake the shrimps until well done.
7. Mix the carrots with the beetroot and the vanilla dressing. Put the salad on a plate and decorate with the shrimps.

Nutritional info:
Calories: 300, Fat: 8g /1.6 tsp
Carbohydrate: 7g, Protein: 10g

FILLED PITA ROLL OR BUN

Serves: 1

Ingredients:
1 stem parsley
50g/3 tbsp cottage cheese
5ml/1 tsp lemon juice
salt
pepper
1 winter carrot
1 pita bun
2 leaves of lettuce
3 slices tomato
4 slices pickle

Instructions:

1. Finely chop the parsley.
2. Mix the parsley with the cottage cheese and lemon juice—flavour with salt and pepper.
3. Grate the carrot.
4. Roast the pita bun until golden brown. Fill the bun with the lettuce, tomato, pickle, cottage cheese and carrot—season with pepper.

Nutritional info:
Calories: 220, Fat: 1g/0.2 tsp
Carbohydrate: 38g, Protein: 13g

SPICY RICE SALAD

Serves: 1

Ingredients:
40g/1.5oz rice
40 ml/1.5oz non-fat yoghurt
0.25 cucumber
60g/2oz cherry tomatoes
100g/4oz corn
1 spring onion
1 stem parsley steel
30g/2 tsp salad dressing
1.2g/0.25 tsp mustard
10ml/2 tsp balsamic vinegar
15ml/1 tbsp milk
salt, pepper to taste

Instructions:
1. Cook the rice as listed on the package.
2. Mix the yoghurt with the dressing, mustard, vinegar and milk and season with salt and pepper.
3. Cut the cucumber lengthwise in half a slice both halves.
4. Cut the tomatoes in half and cut the spring onion into rings.
5. Pour the corn in a colander and leave to drip.
6. Remove the leaves from the parsley stem and finely chop them.
7. Mix the parsley with the vegetables and the sauce with the rice.
8. Season with salt and pepper.

Nutritional info:
Calories: 290, Fat: 7g/1.4 tsp
Carbohydrate: 50g, Protein: 8g

CHOCOLATE CHEESE GRATIN

Serves: 1

Ingredients:
1 small pear
100g/4oz low-fat cream cheese
1 egg yolk
15g/1 tbsp corn starch
5g/1 tsp icing sugar
0.25 lemon/grate and juice
15g/1 tbsp chopped dark chocolate

Instructions:

1. Wash the pear and cut the pear in halve. Remove the core and cut the fruit flesh into thin slices.
2. Stir the egg yolk, corn starch, powder sugar through the cream cheese.
3. Add the grated lemon and the juice of the lemon. Mix thoroughly.
4. Take a small oven form and put the chopped chocolate and cream cheese in it.
5. Press in the pear slices.
6. Put the form in a hot grill until everything is well done.
7. Remove the hot form from the grill and sprinkle chocolate powder on top.

Nutritional info:
Calories: 250, Fat: 8g/1.6 tsp
Carbohydrate: 26g, Protein: 19g

LAYERED SANDWICH

Serves: 1

Ingredients:
1 slice whole-wheat bread
5ml/1 tsp low-fat salad dressing/max 10% fat
2 lettuce leaf
1 tomato
1 slice edamame cheese/max 30% fat
1 slice ham
pepper

Instructions:
1. Smear the dressing onto the slice of bread.
2. Add on top the lettuce, tomato, cheese and ham.
3. Season with enough pepper.

Nutritional info:
Calories: 225, Fat: 7g/1.4 tsp
Carbohydrate: 23g, Protein: 18g

MELON SALAD

Serves: 1

Ingredients:
150g/5oz watermelon
0.13 Cantaloupe melon
0.13 honey melon
2,5g/0.5 tsp ginger powder
30ml/2 tbsp orange juice
7.5ml/1.5 tsp lime juice
15g/ 1 tbsp brown caster sugar

Instructions:
1. Cut each melon type into bite-sized chunks.
2. Mix the orange juice with the lime juice.
3. Add the ginger powder and caster sugar.
4. Add this to the melon chunks in a bowl.
5. Let it rest to soak for about ten minutes.

Nutritional info:
Calories: 190, Fat: 3g /0.6 tsp
Carbohydrate: 35g, Protein: 4g

RADICCHIO SALAD

Serves: 1

Ingredients:
200g/7oz potatoes
10g/1 tbsp pecan nuts
30g/1oz raw ham
1 shallot
5ml/1 tsp oil
1 knife tip sugar
25 ml/2 tbsp vegetable broth
15ml/1 tbsp vinegar
50g/1.5oz radicchio
1 stem parsley steel
25g/1oz gorgonzola cheese

Instructions:
1. Boil the potatoes in their skin until well done.
2. Let them cool, peel them and cut them into slices.
3. Put the slices in a bowl.
4. Chop the pecan nuts and roast them in a dry pan.
5. Bake the ham crisp and then break the ham into pieces.
6. Finely chop the shallot and bake in oil. Stir in the sugar and add the broth and vinegar. Cook this mixture for about 2 minutes and remove the pan from the heat source.
7. Pour this dressing over the potatoes.
8. Finley chops the radicchio and the parsley. Mix both with the pecan nuts and the ham and put into the salad.
9. Break the cheese into little chunks and sprinkle on top of the salad.

Nutritional info:
Calories: 133, Fat: 8g/1.6 tsp
Carbohydrate: 9g, Protein: 5g

MELON TURKEY CROSTINI

Serves: 1

Ingredients:
1 slice whole-wheat bread
some pesto
2 slices turkey salmon
125g/4.5oz sugar melon fruit flesh.

Instructions:
1. Toast the bread and cut the slice in halve. Smear pesto on each halve.
2. Add the turkey salmon.
3. Cut the melon flesh into little chunks and put the melon flesh on top.

Nutritional info:
Calories: 250, Fat: 3g/0.6 tsp
Carbohydrate: 46g, Protein: 20g

TOMATO PASTA

Serves: 1

Ingredients

100g/3.50z whole
wheat pasta
0.5 onion
0.5 garlic clove
125g/4.50z flesh
tomatoes

50g/10z cherry
tomatoes
15ml/1 tbsp oil
balsamic vinegar
salt
pepper

Instructions

1. Cook the pasta as mentioned on the package.
2. Cut the onion and garlic clove into little cubes.
3. Cut the flesh tomatoes into bigger cubes.
4. Heat the oil in a pan.
5. Add the onion, garlic, tomato cubes and the cherry tomatoes. Season this with salt, pepper and balsamic vinegar.
6. Let this simmer until everything is well done.
7. Add the pasta and put everything on a plate.

Nutritional info:
Calories: 460, Fat: 9g/1.8 tsp
Carbohydrate: 79g, Protein: 14g

TOMATO SOUP WITH KALE

Serves: 1

Ingredients:
50g/2oz carrots
50g/2oz of tomato
20g/4 tsp onion
5ml/1 tsp oil
5ml/1 tsp tomato puree
150ml/5oz vegetable broth
25ml/2 tbsp of tomato juice
salt
pepper
1 stem of thyme
15g/1 tbsp of kale
60g/4 tbsp white beans

Instructions:

1. Cut the carrots and tomatoes and onion in cubes.
2. Heat the oil in a pan and add the carrots and onions for about 2-3 minutes. Add the tomatoes and the puree and let this simmer for about 1-2 minutes. Add the broth and the tomato juice.
3. Flavour this with salt, pepper, and the thyme. Put the lid on and cook at a low temperature for about 5 minutes.
4. Add the kale and white beans and cook for 2-3 minutes.

Nutritional info:
Calories: 380, Fat: 5g/1 tsp
Carbohydrate: 58g, Protein: 26g

IN-BETWEEN

CRISP BREAD WITH MUSTARD

Serves: 1

Ingredients:
1 crispbread
some mustard

Instructions:
1.   Smear the crispbread with some mustard.

Nutritional info:
Calories: 30, Fat: 0.4g/1.8 tsp
Carbohydrates: 6g, Protein: 1g

CRISPY YOGHURT

Serves: 1

Ingredients:
15g/1 tsp of almond flakes
50g/2oz mixed berries
180g/6oz low-fat yoghurt
60g/5 tbsp spring water
grated lemon peel
30g/2 tbsp lemon juice
half a piece of crispbread

Instructions:
1. Heat the almond flakes in a pan without butter, let it out of the pan and allow to cool.
2. Wash the berries and let them dry.
3. Mix the yoghurt with the spring water, grated lemon peel and lemon juice.
4. Add the berries and mix.
5. Sprinkle the crispbread and garnish the yoghurt, add the almond flakes.

Nutritional info:
Calories: 142, Fat: 6g/1.2 tsp
Carbohydrates: 16g, Protein: 28g

CUCUMBER COTTAGE CHEESE

Serves: 1

Ingredients:
1 small cucumber
30g/2 tbsp non-fat cottage cheese
dill
salt
pepper

Instructions:
1. Cut the cucumber in halves on the long side and remove the core with a spoon.
2. Add a little bit of dill, salt, and pepper to the cottage cheese
3. Put this mixture in the empty cores of the cucumber.

Nutritional info:
Calories: 50, Fat: 0g
Carbohydrates: 6g, Protein: 7g

CHICORY HAM ROLLS

Serves: 1

Ingredients:
2 spring onions
100g/4oz low fat cream cheese
4 slices boiled ham
4 leaves chicory

Instructions:
1. Chop the spring onions
2. Add the onions to the cream cheese and blend well.
3. Put one chicory leaf on each ham slice.
4. Divide the cream cheese mixture on top.
5. Roll up the ham slices.

Nutritional info:
Calories: 250, Fat: 4g/0.8 tsp
Carbohydrates: 10g, Protein: 27g

FRUIT CURD DESSERT

Serves: **1**

Ingredients:
2,5 apricots
50g/2oz grapes
200g/7oz lean curd
30ml/2 tbsp of skimmed milk
5ml/1 tsp of lemon juice

Instructions:
1. Cut the apricots into slices and wash and halve the grapes.
2. Bring the curd with the milk and flavour the lemon juice.
3. Mix most of the fruit with the curd.
4. Make the mixture in a bowl and the rest of the fruit on top for decoration.

Nutritional info:
Calories: 179, Fat: 1g/0.2 tsp
Carbohydrates: 12g, Protein: 28g

HONEY MUSTARD SAUCE

Serves: 10-12 portions

Ingredients:
200g/7oz mustard
150ml/5oz honey
salt
pepper

Instructions:
1. Mix the honey with the mustard and season with
    salt and pepper.

Nutritional info:
Calories: 60, Fat: 1g/0.2 tsp
Carbohydrates: 11g, Protein: 1g
108

KEFIR STRAWBERRY DAIQUIRI

Serves: 1

Ingredients:
some sugar
200g/7oz strawberries
15g/1 tbsp vanilla sugar
30ml/2 tbsp lime juice
250g/9oz kefir

Instructions:
1. Dip the rim of a glass into the lime juice first than in the sugar.
2. Puree the strawberries with vanilla sugar and lime juice.
3. Stir in the kefir.
4. Fill the glass.

Nutritional info:
Calories: 240, Fat: 4g/0.8 tsp
Carbohydrates: 42g, Protein: 10g

OAT CLAY COTTAGE CHEESE

Serves: 1

Ingredients:
200g/7oz low-fat cottage cheese
80g/3oz cream cheese
5g/1 tsp sweetener
60g/4 tbsp oat clay
some lemon juice

Instructions:
1. Mix the cottage cheese, cream cheese and sweetener and blend well.
2. Solve the oat clay in some water and stir into the mixture.
3. Season to taste with the lemon juice.

Nutritional info:
Calories: 350, Fat: 5g/1 tsp
Carbohydrates: 28g, Protein: 46g

MELON CUCUMBER SNACK

Serves: 1

Ingredients:
120g/4.5oz watermelon flesh
80g/3oz peeled cucumber
2-3 leaf mint

Instructions:
1. Cut the melon flesh and cucumber into little cubes.
2. Mix in a bowl.
3. Garnish with the mint.

Nutritional info:
Calories: 50, Fat: 0g
Carbohydrates: 12g, Protein: 1g

PAPAYA WITH COTTAGE CHEESE

Serves: 1

Ingredients:
100g/4oz papaya
200g/7oz cottage cheese
2 stalks of lemon balm
15ml/1 tbsp of spring water
15ml/1 tbsp of lemon juice

Instructions:
1. Cut the papaya into small cubes and stir into the cottage cheese.
2. Wipe and cut the lemon balm leaves. These freshly cut leaves mix me with the spring water and lemon juice.
3. Then stir into the cottage cheese

Nutritional info:
Calories: 220, Fat: 9g/1.8 tsp
Carbohydrates: 6g, Protein: 27g

TOMATO WITH CREAM CHEESE

Serves: 1

Ingredients:
2 tomatoes
30g/2 tbsp low-fat cream cheese
various herbs

Instructions:
1. Cut each tomato in halves and remove the flesh.
2. Fill the tomato with the cream cheese.
3. Season with the herbs.

Nutritional info:
Calories: 65, Fat: 2g/0.4 tsp
Carbohydrates: 4g, Protein: 7g

TOMATO MELON BOWL

Serves: 1

Ingredients:
200g/7oz sugar melon
5g/1 tsp chopped basil
300ml/10oz tomato juice
75g/3oz chicken breast fillet
1 slice crispbread
pepper
tabasco

Instructions:
1. Cut about 50g/2.5oz of the melon flesh into cubes.
2. Put this in a bowl and add the basil.
3. Blend the remaining melon fruit flesh and add the tomato juice—season with pepper and tabasco.
4. Add the flesh cubes and mix.
5. Cut the chicken breast fillet into stripes and garnish the mixture.
6. Eat this with the crispbread slice.

Nutritional info:
Calories: 250, Fat: 2g/0.4 tsp
Carbohydrates: 40g, Protein: 19g

YOGHURT WITH WALNUTS

Serves: 1

Ingredients:
100g/3.5oz yoghurt
2 walnuts
sweetener

Instructions:
1. Break the walnuts into halves and mix them with the yoghurt.
2. Add sweetener to taste.

Nutritional info:
Calories: 95, Fat: 6g/1.2 tsp
Carbohydrates: 5g, Protein: 5g

DINNER

POTATO SAUERKRAUT OVEN

Serves: 1

Ingredients:
300g/10oz potatoes
200g/7oz sauerkraut
0.5 apple
5g/1 tsp dried cranberries
5g/1 tsp almond leaves
2.5ml/0.5 tsp honey

Instructions:

1. Peel the potatoes and cut them into little cubes. Cook them well done in about 15 minutes.
2. Put the sauerkraut in a sieve and let it drain as much as possible.
3. Cut the apple into little cubes.
4. Mix the cooked potatoes with the sauerkraut and the apple cubes.
5. Put this mixture in an oven dish.
6. Sprinkle the almond leaves on top and drizzle with honey.
7. Bake in a hot oven until golden brown. Gas mark 6

Nutritional info:
Calories: 350, Fat: 6g/1.2 tsp
Carbohydrates: 59g, Protein: 10g

POTATOES WITH A SALT CRUST

Serves: 1

Ingredients:
250 g/9oz small solid potatoes
22,5g/1.5 tbsp coarse sea salt
100g/3.5oz low fat cream cheese
various herbs by choice

Instructions:

1. Put the potatoes with the peel in a pan and fill the pan with water until half full.
2. Add sea salt on top.
3. Place a tea towel between the lid and the pan and cook this way the potatoes well done.
4. Drain the potatoes when they are well cooked but leave a layer of water in the pan.
5. Recook the potatoes till all water evaporates. The potatoes begin to shrink.
6. Put the shrunken potatoes on a plate and add the cream cheese. Garnish by choice with herbs like parsley.

Nutritional info:
Calories: 255, Fat: 6g/1.2 tsp
Carbohydrates: 41g, Protein: 19g

MASHED POTATOES PEES

Serves: 1

Ingredients:
175g/6oz potatoes
75g/3oz frozen peas
1 stem lemon steel
60ml/4 tbsp milk
8g/1.5 tsp margarine
salt
pepper

Instructions:
1. Peel the potatoes and cut them into four pieces. Cook them until ready.
2. Add the peas about 5 minutes before the potatoes are fully cooked.
3. Rinse the potatoes and peas and mash both with milk and margarine.
4. Chop the lemon
5. Mix the lemon with the mash and season the mash with salt and pepper.

Nutritional info:
Calories: 250, Fat: 9g/1.8 tsp
Carbohydrates: 33g, Protein: 9g

MASHED POTATOES TOMATOES

Serves: 1

Ingredients:
250g/9oz potatoes
1 stem basil
60ml/4 tbsp milk
15g/1 tbsp tomato paste
8g/1.5 tsp margarine

Instructions:

1. Cook the potatoes until fully cooked.
2. Rinse them and mash them with milk, tomato paste and margarine.
3. Finely tear the basil stem and mix this with the potato mash. If necessary season with salt and pepper.

Nutritional info:

Calories: 250, Fat: 9g/1.8 tsp
Carbohydrates: 35g, Protein: 7g

MASHED POTATOES CARROTS

Serves: 1

Ingredients:
150g/5oz potatoes
100g/3.5oz carrots
1 stem chervil
60ml/4 tbsp milk
8g/1.5 tsp
pepper

Instructions:

1. Cut the potatoes and the carrots into little cubes. Cook them together in a pan until fully cooked. Rinse and add the milk and margarine and mix everything to a mash.
2. Chop the chervil and mix into the puree—season with salt and pepper.

Nutritional info:
Calories: 200, Fat: 9g/1.8 tsp
Carbohydrates: 25g, Protein: 5g

PINEAPPLE STEW

Serves: 1

Ingredients:
40g/2.5 tbsp whole wheat rice
2 spring onions
4 cherry tomatoes
2 canned pineapple rings
100g/3.50z chicken escalope
salt
pepper
15ml/1 tbsp sour cream
45ml/3 tbsp pineapple juice
oil
water

Instructions:

1. Cook the rice as described on the package.
2. Finely chop the onions and cut the tomatoes in halve.
3. Cut the pineapple rings into pieces.
4. Cut the chicken flesh into stripes.
5. Bake the chicken strips in a non-stick frying pan with a little oil.
6. Season with salt and pepper.
7. When the chicken strips cooked well done, remove the flesh from the pan.
8. Put the spring onion in the pan and slowly bake the onion. Add the pineapple pieces with the juice and a little bit of water.
9. Let it cook and then add the cream. Add the meat and reheat. Do not recook, just warm up.
10. Put the meat and the boiled rice on a plate.

Nutritional info:
Calories: 400, Fat: 8g/1.6 tsp
Carbohydrates: 53g, Protein: 29g

ASPARAGUS TOMATO SALAD

Serves: 1

Ingredients:
100g/3.50z white asparagus
100g/3.50z cherry tomatoes
25g/1.5 tbsp mixed salad
3 stems chives
5ml/1 tsp honey
5ml/1 tsp vinegar
5g/1 tsp mustard
5ml/1 tsp oil
salt
pepper

Instructions:

1. Cut the ends of the asparagus and slice the asparagus into little pieces.
2. Cook the asparagus for about 8 minutes until just soft.
3. Cut the cherry tomatoes into halves and finely chop the chives.
4. Mix the honey with the vinegar, mustard, some salt and pepper. Stir in the oil.
5. Mix this dressing with the asparagus, tomatoes and mixed salad.

Nutritional info:

Calories: 160, Fat: 10g/2 tsp
Carbohydrates: 13g, Protein: 3g

STRAWBERRY CHICKEN

Serves: 1

Ingredients:
250g/4.5oz strawberries,
25g/2 tbsp shallot
10ml/2 tsp oil
15g/1 tbsp green pepper
15ml/1 tbsp vinegar
2.5ml/0.5 tsp honey
salt
150g/5oz chicken fillet
2 baguette slices

Instructions:
1. Cut the strawberries into quarters.
2. Cut the shallot into rings. Heat the oil and gently stir fry the shallot until the shallot is soft and a little bit brown.
3. Add the strawberries and pepper.
4. Cool off with vinegar, stir in the honey, season with the salt and green pepper.
5. Season the fillet and stir fry the meat in the oil until light brown. Slice the meat and add the chutney and baguette slices on a plate.

Nutritional info:
Calories: 230, Fat: 10g/2 tsp
Carbohydrates: 25g, Protein: 37g

BELL PEPPER CHICKEN

Serves: 1

Ingredients:
150g/5oz potatoes
1 red bell pepper
200g/7oz sauerkraut
125g/4.5oz broth
5g/1 tsp paprika
100g/3.5oz chicken breast fillet
5 ml/1 tsp oil
30ml/2 tbsp low-fat milk

Instructions:

1. Thoroughly cook the potatoes.
2. Cut the bell pepper into strips.
3. Heat the broth and add the bell pepper stripes and the sauerkraut.
4. Let this mixture stew until the vegetables are well done.
5. Heat oil in a baking pan and bake the chicken breast fillet.
6. Rinse the potatoes, heat some milk and pour the milk with the potatoes and mash.
7. Put everything on a plate.

Nutritional info:
Calories: 385, Fat: 10g/2 tsp
Carbohydrates: 36g, Protein: 36g

CREOLE PAN

Serves: 1

Ingredients:
2 spring onions
40g/2.5 tbsp whole wheat rice
2 ml/0.2 tsp tomato juice
salt
pepper
1 small bay leaf
1 pinch clove powder
125g/4.5oz bell pepper
100g/3.5oz zucchini
75g/3oz sugar melon
40g/1.5oz low-fat ham chunks

Instructions:

1. Cut the spring onion into little pieces, add the rice and shortly fry in a non-stick pan. Cool down with the tomato juice.
2. Season with salt, pepper, and the bay leaf.
3. Cut the bell pepper and the courgette into little cubes and add in the pan. Put a lid on the pan and let everything cook until well done. Stir now and then.
4. Cut the sugar melon flesh into cubes and add in the pan. Cook it until the melon flesh is as warm as the rest.
5. Put the mixture on a plate and garnish with the ham chunks.

Nutritional info:
Calories: 300, Fat: 4g/0.8 tsp
Carbohydrates: 51g, Protein: 17g

HOT CHINESE NOODLES

Serves: 1

Ingredients:
50g/2oz Chinese noodles
50g/2oz carrots
50g/2oz green beans
50g/2oz cauliflower
50g/2oz broccoli
125g/4oz chicken breast
5g/1 tsp oil
1 shallot
some ginger
soy sauce
chilli sauce
lime juice

Instructions:

1. Cook the Chinese noodles as described on the package, let them cool down quickly.
2. Peel or wash the carrots, green beans, cauliflower and broccoli. Chop everything into little pieces and cook in salted water until semi-cooked.
3. Cut the chicken breast into strips and chop the shallot. Heat the oil in a non-stick frying pan and fry the shallot with the ginger. Add the meat and the vegetables and stir fry until semi-cooked.
4. Season with soy sauce, chilli sauce, and lime juice.

Nutritional info:
Calories: 390, Fat: 8g/1.6 tsp
Carbohydrates: 30g, Protein: 39g

PASTA PAN

Serves: 1

Ingredients:
100g/3.5oz pasta
salt
0.5 garlic clove
40g/1.5oz cherry tomatoes
1 leek
4 shrimps/unpeeled
2 tsp oil divided
pepper
50 ml/2oz broth
some sugar

Instructions:
1. Cook the pasta as described on the package.
2. Slice the garlic, cut the tomatoes into halves and the leek into rings.
3. Thoroughly peel the shrimps and remove the colon.
4. Bake the shrimps in one tsp of oil for about two minutes.
5. Add the garlic and bake for another minute— season with salt and pepper.
6. Remove the shrimps from the pan.
7. Add the tomato pieces and the leek rings and bake until both are somewhat soft.
8. Rinse the pasta and add the pasta to the tomato and leek.
9. Add one tsp of oil and bake until warm. Cool off with the broth.
10. Add the shrimps, mix everything thoroughly and recook. Season with salt and pepper and put everything on a plate.

Nutritional info:
Calories: 470, Fat: 6g/1.2 tsp
Carbohydrates: 76g, Protein: 31g

PEPPER FISH WITH LENTILS

Serves: 1

Ingredients:
50g/2oz red lentils
200g/7oz tomato cubes
125g/4.5oz cod fillet
175 ml/6oz vegetable stock
1 onion
1 garlic clove
5ml/1 tsp olive oil
pepper
cayenne pepper

Instructions:

1. Dice the onion and the garlic clove.
2. Heat the olive oil in a pan and heat the onion and garlic.
3. Rinse the red lentils and add these with the onion and garlic in the pan.
4. Add the stock and put a lit on the pan.
5. Let this cook for about 8 minutes.
6. Add the tomato cubes and season with cayenne pepper.
7. Rub the cod fillet with pepper and slice the fish into cubes.
8. Mix with the lentils in the pan and let it simmer for about 5 minutes.

Nutritional info:
Calories: 130, Fat: 7g/1.4 tsp
Carbohydrates: 31g, Protein: 35g

POTATOES HERBAL CHEESE

Serves: 1

Ingredients:
150g/5oz potatoes
1 egg
75g/3oz cream cheese
1 bunch mixed herbs
15ml/1 tbsp milk
salt
pepper

Instructions:
1. Cook the potatoes for about 20 minutes till soft.
2. Boil the egg for about 10 minutes, cool off with cold water and peel the egg.
3. Finely chop the mixed herbs and stir into the cream cheese.
4. Mix the milk, salt and pepper and stir through the cream cheese.
5. Cut the boiled egg into cubes and stir through the cream cheese.
6. Put the potatoes on a plate and add the cream cheese.

Nutritional info:
Calories: 260, Fat: 7g/1.4 tsp
Carbohydrates: 25g, Protein: 21g

POTATOES PEPPER CHEESE

Serves: 1

Ingredients:
200g/7oz low-fat cream cheese
200g/7oz potatoes unpeeled
mineral water
1 onion
1 stem chives
15g/3 tsp green pepper
salt

Instructions:

1. Cook the potatoes in their skin until done.
2. Mix the water and the cream cheese and stir until you have a creamy mass.
3. Finely slice the onion, make rolls of the chives and stir both; add pepper into the cream mass.
4. Season with a little bit of salt.
5. Put the skinned potatoes on a plate and put the cream mass next to it.

Nutritional info:

Calories: 349, Fat: 9g/1.8 tsp
Carbohydrates: 39g, Protein: 26g,

BEEF WITH RADISHES

Serves: 1

Ingredients:
70g/3oz steak
salt
pepper
2.5g/0.5 tsp mustard
2.5g/0.5 tsp sugar
5ml/1 tsp broth
15ml/1 tbsp lemon juice
10ml/2 tsp oil
1 spring onion
4 radishes
2 stems parsley

Instructions:

1. Season the steak with salt and pepper. Put one tsp of oil in a pan and bake the steak well done
2. Mix the mustard with the sugar, the broth, lime juice and the rest of the oil.
3. Finely cut the spring onion and chop the radishes and parsley.
4. Mix everything thoroughly.
5. Slice the steak and put the slices on a plate.
6. Garnish with the onion mixture and drizzle the mustard sauce on top.

Nutritional info:
Calories: 230, Fat: 9g/1.8 tsp
Carbohydrates: 4g, Protein: 33g

BLUEBERRIES ESCALOPE

Serves: 1

Ingredients:
150g/5oz potatoes
160g/5oz escalope
salt
pepper
15ml/1 tbsp oil
45ml/3 tbsp water
5ml/1 tsp instant vegetable broth
5ml/1 tsp light balsamic vinegar
100g/3.5oz blueberries.

Instructions:

1. Cook the potatoes and in the meantime season the escalope with salt and pepper.
2. Heat the oil in a non-stick frying pan and bake the escalope golden brown on both sides.
3. Remove the escalope from the pan and keep the escalope warm.
4. Add the water in the frying pan and the instant broth and stir until there is a smooth mixture.
5. Add the vinegar and stir in the blueberries. Heat everything and season with salt and pepper.
6. Take a plate and put the potatoes and the escalope on it. Add the blueberry sauce on top.

Nutritional info:

Calories: 345, Fat: 8g/1.6 tsp
Carbohydrates: 31g, Protein: 37

PORK FILLET WITH MELON

Serves: 1

Ingredients:
40g/2oz whole wheat parboiled rice
1 small onion
1 small red or yellow bell pepper
75g/3oz sugar melon
15ml/1 tbsp apple vinegar
salt
pepper
7.5ml/1.5 tsp oil
2 pork fillet medallions each 75g/2.5oz
thyme

Instructions:

1. Cook the rice as described on the package.
2. Peel the onion and cut the onion into rings. Wash the bell pepper and cut it into fine strips.
3. Cut the flesh of the sugar melon into little pieces. Mix the melon pieces with the onion and the bell pepper.
4. Mix the vinegar with the oil and some salt and pepper. Drizzle this over the salad.
5. Add half a tsp of oil in a non-stick frying pan and bake the medallions until crispy brown on both sides—season with salt, pepper and thyme.
6. Drain the rice.
7. Put the medallions on a plate together with the salad and the rice.

Nutritional info:
Calories: 300, Fat: 6g/1.2 tsp
Carbohydrates: 44g, Protein: 20g

SALMON IN CURRY

Serves: 1

Ingredients:
300g/10oz salmon fillet
250 ml/9oz vegetable broth
200g/7oz broccoli
salt
1 onion
5 ml/1 tsp oil
50 ml/3 tbsp vegetable broth
1 egg yolk
curry powder

Instructions:

1. Cook the salmon fillet in the 250 ml broth until the fillet is well-done.
2. Cook the broccoli in water.
3. Finely chop one onion. Heat 1 tsp of oil in a pan, and heat the chopped onion. Add 50 ml of broth to cool down the onion.
4. Mix the yolk with some of the broth, add to the pan and stir in to thicken the mass—season with the curry powder.
5. Put the fillet and the broccoli on a plate and pour the sauce on top.

Nutritional info:
Calories: 410, Fat: 9g/1.8 tsp
Carbohydrates: 15g, Protein: 65g

NOTES

NOTES

NOTES

Made in the USA
Columbia, SC
30 March 2021